Psychotherapy in
the Future

Committee on Therapy
Group for the Advancement of Psychiatry

Allen D. Rosenblatt, La Jolla, CA, Chairperson
Gerald Adler, Boston, MA
Jules R. Bemporad, Boston, MA
Eugene B. Feigelson, Brooklyn, NY
Robert Michels, New York, NY
Andrew P. Morrison, Cambridge, MA
William C. Offenkrantz, Carefree, AZ

Psychotherapy in the Future

Formulated by the Committee on Therapy
Group for the Advancement of Psychiatry

Report No. 133

Published by

American Psychiatric Press, Inc.

Washington, DC
London, England

Copyright ©1992 Group for the Advancement of Psychiatry.
ALL RIGHTS RESERVED
Manufactured in the United States of America on acid-free paper.
94 93 92 91 4 3 2 1
Published by American Psychiatric Press, Inc., 1400 K Street, N.W.,
Washington, DC 20005.

Library of Congress Cataloging-in-Publication Data

Psychotherapy in the future/formulated by the Committee on Therapy, Group for the Advancement of Psychiatry
    p. cm. -- (Report ; no. 133)
    Includes bibliographical references
    ISBN 0-87318-201-4 (alk. paper)
    1. Psychotherapy--United States--Forecasting. 2. Twenty-first cen-
tury--Forecasts. I. Group for the Advancement of Psychiatry. Committee on Therapy. II. Series: Report (Group for the Advancement of
Psychiatry : 1984) ; no. 133.
    [DNLM: 1. Managed Care Programs--trends--United States.
2. Mental Health Services--trends--United States. 3. Psychother-
apy--trends--United States. 4. Socioeconomic Factors. W1 RE209BR
no. 133 / WN 420 P97565]
RC321.G7 no. 133
[RC480.5]
616.89 s--dc20
[616.89'14'0112]
DNLM/DLC
for Library of Congress   91-21996
                                                             CIP

British Cataloguing in Publication Data

A CIP record is available from the British Library.

Contents

Introduction

Psychiatry, with its special ties to both the biological and social worlds, has been particularly responsive to the social, economic, and political forces that are so dramatically changing the face of medical practice. The practice of psychotherapy, once the most dominant aspect of psychiatric practice, is perhaps the most vulnerable of all areas to these pressures; and concern has been expressed that the physician psychotherapist will soon become an endangered species.

In an earlier publication (GAP Committee on Therapy 1986), we explored the impact of socioeconomic changes on the teaching of psychotherapy and its implications for practice. We now intend to examine current trends for their effect both on the practitioner and on the practice of psychotherapy in an attempt to understand who will practice psychotherapy a generation from now and what that practice will be like. When we speak of psychotherapy, we refer to both long-term and short-term psychotherapy, still the primary activity of practicing psychiatrists (whether or not it is combined with medication). However, as will become clear, we believe that long-term exploratory psychotherapy will be the most significantly affected of the psychotherapeutic modalities. Long-term supportive care, under the rubric of "medical case management," will probably continue to be available to some degree. Our attempt to predict the future of these various modalities of psychotherapy does not imply any comparative evaluation of their merits, when appropriately applied.

However, we *do* assume the therapeutic efficacy of long-term psychotherapy in appropriate cases.

Forecasting the future is always risky, yet the attempt is necessary for any individual or societal adaptation to a changing world. In our exploration of the issues, we may well overestimate the importance of some trends and miss the significance of others. The justification for our endeavor is not any pretension of omniscient prophecy, but the urgent wish to call attention to the probable results of certain observable trends. If these results appear to be undesirable or even intolerable, then efforts should be made either to alter the trends or to adapt to the inevitable.

Whether the changes we predict are to be considered "good" or "bad" depends on the answer to the question, "Good for whom?" From the standpoint of the practitioners, many of the changes forecast will limit their ability to practice the way they desire. On the other hand, from the standpoint of those consumers who have hitherto been unable to afford *any* psychiatric treatment, limited psychiatric benefits will be more widely available. Thus there are legitimate conflicts between public health needs, needs of individual patients, and the autonomy of the psychotherapist.

We will address the issues of what the practice and practitioner of psychotherapy will be in the next generation within the framework of three questions: 1) Who will provide the service? 2) How will the service be provided? and 3) What will the service consist of? We will then examine some possible solutions to problems generated by this future scenario.

Chapter 1

Who Will Provide the Service?

The Demedicalization of Psychotherapy

Over the past 30 years there has been a steady increase in absolute as well as relative numbers of nonpsychiatrist psychotherapists (GAP 1987; Manderscheid and Barrett 1987). By the mid-1970s the number of psychiatrists in the United States about equaled the number of clinical social workers, and each were almost twice the number of clinical psychologists. In the subsequent 15 years, clinical psychologists and clinical social workers each almost tripled their numbers, while the number of psychiatrists grew by less than 40%. As a result of these trends, clinical psychologists now outnumber psychiatrists, and clinical social workers now outnumber either psychiatrists or clinical psychologists by two to one (Goleman 1990; Manderscheid and Barrett 1987). In addition, there are large undocumented numbers of nonmedical psychotherapists who are from none of the above disciplines. Psychotherapy already has become a predominantly nonmedical activity, and there is every indication that this trend will continue until eventually the medically trained psychotherapist becomes rare.

Several factors appear to be involved in this change. The quality of training of nonmedical professionals has been greatly enhanced by the establishment of more and more freestanding clinical training programs for psychologists and for social workers, the two most numerous categories of nonmedical therapists. Moreover, both of these professional groups have become increasingly sophisticated, both politically and economically. They have obtained parity with medical therapists in several critical areas, such as insurance reimbursement, admitting privileges for psychologists in psychiatric hospitals in some states, and admission to full clinical psychoanalytic training. Thus, those who have selected psychotherapy as a career no longer need to undergo arduous medical training as the preferred route to their chosen career. In fact, the increasing emphasis on biology in psychiatric training may result in potential medical psychotherapists pursuing other mental health disciplines, further decreasing the numbers of such individuals in psychiatry (Feigelson and Friedman 1984).

Even now, because of their improved training in psychotherapy, psychologists and psychiatric social workers are more likely than before to work psychotherapeutically with the psychological problems of severely disturbed patients. In contrast, psychiatrists, with their increasingly biological orientation, are more likely to emphasize the use of psychopharmacological agents.

On the other hand, the growing differentiation and subspecialization within psychiatry have led to a decrease in the numbers of psychiatrists who elect to obtain advanced training in psychotherapy and to practice it. When psychiatrists were asked in a recent survey to rank the importance of various skills in their profession, skills in psychotherapy were "notably reduced in the ranking of their importance" compared to a similar survey taken years previously (Langsley and Yager 1988). These authors concluded that, whereas "it has been estimated that 70% of psychiatric time used to be devoted to office psychotherapy for personality disorders and neurotic inhibitions . . . long-term therapy and treatment aimed at overcoming problems that diminish the quality of life have given way to treatment for serious psychotic disorders. . . . Threats to life and functioning are deemed the only reasons for treatment. . . . The shift in caseload to the more seriously ill has been a consequence of cost containment and changed third-party coverage of psychiatric services" (p. 473). Thus, as nonpsychiatrists do more and more psychotherapy, psychiatrists do less and less psychotherapy.

There are also many nonpsychiatrist physicians who practice and bill for psychotherapy. Their current and future impact on the overall practice of psychotherapy is unclear; however, in Canada, as physician office visits have decreased, billings for one-hour psychotherapy by such nonpsychiatrist physicians have increased (Richmond and Brown 1980). This experience suggests that nonpsychiatrist physicians may tend to practice (or at least bill for) psychotherapy as a response to falling practice income. A similar phenomenon seems to have been occurring in this country. A study of CHAMPUS utilization data revealed that not only had psychiatrists' share of the market for outpatient behavioral health visits dropped from 36% to 21% from 1982 to 1987, but the percentage of such visits by attending physicians had more than doubled, from 5.6% to 11.5% (Open Minds, April 11, 1990).

It is likely that psychiatrists will continue to be the most *expensive* mental health professionals who conduct psychotherapy. In Massachusetts the hourly fee for a psychiatrist averages about $10 more than that for a psychologist and about $25 more than that for a social worker (Dezell 1988). Nationally, the median fee for psychiatrists in private practice was estimated in 1985 to be $90 per session, while clinical psychologists averaged $65 per session, and social workers averaged $50 per session (Goleman 1985). In addition to caring for the financially elite, psychiatrists will therefore be expected to do those things that are most critical (for example, treatment planning, supervision, and evaluation) that are perceived (correctly or incorrectly) as most dangerous (such as ECT), or that require medical training (for example, prescribing medication). Psychotherapy is none of these.

One factor, however, may weaken this trend toward demedicalization. If the current surplus of physicians continues to increase, a reduction in the disparity between medical and nonmedical fees may result, with a concomitant diminution of pressure to use physicians' time in a most cost efficient manner. In the presence of a continuing or increasing demand for psychotherapy, there will be physicians (both psychiatrists and nonpsychiatrists) willing to practice it, even at lower remuneration. Nevertheless, a higher level of reimbursement for psychopharmacologists may encourage potential medical psychotherapists to gravitate instead toward more biological treatment modalities. Even so, the physician psychotherapist will probably grow increasingly apart from other nonpsychotherapist physicians. The social worker, psychologist, and physician who practice psychotherapy already have more in common with each other, in terms of professional identity, than they have in common with their nonpsychotherapist colleagues.

It is possible, then, that out of this continuing subspecialization in psychotherapy by both medical and nonmedical professions, a new mental health profession will emerge—that of psychotherapy, with psychoanalysis as a subspecialty. This new profession will draw practitioners from varied medical and nonmedical backgrounds, united by a common interest and training in psychotherapy and, for some, advanced training in psychoanalysis. Lawrence Kubie, a generation ahead of his time, made a proposal similar to our prediction in 1957, but the time was not then ripe for its implementation.

The major consequence of such a differentiation of psychotherapy from medicine and psychiatry will be the imposition of an even greater strain on the medical identity of the medically trained psychotherapist. This issue will be further examined in a later section.

The Gender of Psychotherapists

One consequence of the demedicalization of psychotherapy has been a shift in its gender ratio. Psychiatric social workers and nurses, both increasing in numbers, are predominantly female, and women account for approximately 30% of psychologists practicing psychotherapy (Directory of the American Psychological Association 1989), a larger proportion than is the case for their physician counterparts. However, the feminization of psychotherapy that has resulted from the mushrooming of nonmedical therapists has been reflected also within psychiatry.

There are more than 80,000 female physicians in the United States and an additional 19,000 female residents (Baker 1987). The number of female physicians has been steadily rising, from 7% of all physicians in 1967 to 14% in 1985 and will continue to rise for some time. More than a third of the current medical students are women (Bickel 1988), and the proportion of female medical students has been rising 1% per year since 1974. Three-fourths of these female physicians provide direct patient care, and almost 70% of female medical students choose primary care specialties or psychiatry.

The same pattern is reflected in psychiatry. In 1985, only 19% of psychiatrists were women, but 38% of all psychiatry residents and almost 50% of child psychiatry residents were women (Association of American Medical Colleges 1987).

Compared with their male counterparts, female physicians are more likely to 1) be younger (73% are under age 40, understandable with the rapid recent increase in women medical students), 2) hold a salaried position, 3) earn less money in private practice, 4) be sued less often, 5) see more female patients, and 6) be less involved in organized medicine, including board certification (Fenton et al. 1987).

Already, in many parts of the western world, the majority of physicians are women. In this country although the proportion and absolute number of women in medicine are increasing, the consequences of these increases are less clear. The historic consequences of the feminization of any vocation or profession have been a reduction in status and reduction in earning power in that area. Since, at least currently, these women in medicine and psychiatry are young, tend not to seek involvement in organized medicine, and tend to work in primary care areas, they may be subject to similar economic exploitation, especially in a managed health care setting. It remains to be seen if the concomitant rapid equalization of women's rights and status will neutralize this historic reduction in earnings.

We may see a phenomenon similar to that which happened in the field of teaching in this country, originally a male profession. As more women entered the field, the number of men decreased, particularly in the elementary and secondary schools (Arnold 1985), so that women now provide most of the direct teaching. However, it is still the exception for a principal or superintendent to be female, even though there is a large pool of qualified women from which to draw.

If the same scenario holds true for medicine, primary care would be provided cheaply by women, while tertiary care would be referred to specialists who would probably be male. Policy making would still be done almost exclusively by men at the upper administrative levels. This transformation would affect the income not only of women physicians but of most primary care physicians. Government and the insurance industry have already set the precedent of devaluing noninvasive or "cognitive" procedures, while invasive procedures continue to command large payments. An hour of psychotherapy is reimbursed at a much lower rate than a 15 minute cervical dilatation and uterine curettage. The Harvard study by Hsiao et al. (1988), proposing a resource-based relative value scale (RBRVS) of medical fees for Medicare (and enacted by Congress in the Physician Reform Act of 1989), represents a step toward some correction of these disparities. Nevertheless, it is unlikely that they will be eliminated. At the time of this writing, psychotherapy services by psychiatrists do not appear to be significantly benefited by the recommendations of the Harvard study. (Proposals are under consideration to provide increments of reimbursement based on the dangerousness of the patient or the suicidal risk involved or the number of family members seen in consultation, rather than the complexity or depth of the psychotherapy required.)

The pooling of women in the primary care areas provides a work force that could accelerate the trend toward wide discrepancies in payment between invasive and noninvasive care and therefore increase discrepancies in income between physicians in various fields. In the future, primary care, including psychotherapy, may be a service provided mostly by women at low cost, while the more lucrative and prestigious tertiary care and invasive procedures may be provided mostly by men.

On the other hand, a pool of women providing primary care may benefit patients, as well as decrease costs of providing health care. One of the purposes of capitation fees (given to medical schools by the federal government to encourage larger medical school classes) was to increase the number of physicians available for primary care of underserved populations. To date, the consequent greater numbers of physicians have not decreased the cost of health care, and there are still large underserved groups in the population, such as the chronically mentally ill. It is conceivable that increasing numbers of women physicians will provide a work force that meets the needs of these patients at a lower cost, although noneconomic factors, such as individual interest and commitment, will play the major role.

Aside from individual interest, a female physician's choice to practice in primary care and psychotherapy could be influenced by the lack of female role models in higher ranking positions, including those in academia. Bickel (1988) reports that, for the cohort of physicians first appointed in 1976 to medical school faculties, 12% of men but only 3% of women had been promoted to the rank of professor by 1987.

These trends in part result from the current tendency of women to be less prolific in research than their male counterparts (Bickel 1988). At a time when the proportion of women in the field is increasing, this differential may be cause for concern, foreshadowing a future diminution of research productivity in the field.

As the number of women in psychiatry increases, more women are talking about and writing about their experiences, both as women and as professionals. These contributions are having a positive effect on the theory and practice of psychotherapy. Women have historically played a stronger role in psychoanalysis than in other areas of medicine. Indeed, some female psychoanalysts (for example, Frieda Fromm-Reichmann and Karen Horney) vigorously questioned and modified Freud's ideas on the psychology of women. However, until recently, there was limited social support for women to energetically explore revisions in theories regarding women.

As more peers have become available for dialogue and less of their energy is needed to defend their roles against prejudice, women's productivity is increasing; they are writing more and becoming progressively more involved in the politics of the psychiatric profession. As of this writing, The American Psychiatric Association and Group for the Advancement of Psychiatry have women as presidents, as has the American Psychoanalytic Association on several occasions in the past. A voluminous body of literature about the psychology and psychopathology of women has grown rapidly since the mid-1960s, much of it written by female psychiatrists. In the coming years, the role of women in shaping the future of psychiatry and thus partially shaping psychotherapy, both in theory and practice, will probably continue to increase in importance.

Chapter 2

How Will the Service
Be Provided?

Trends Toward Managed Health Care

We are in the midst of a revolution in the provision of health care that started some 20 years ago. The traditional model of individual practitioners providing fee-for-service medical care is being replaced by a variety of ever larger groups, contracting to provide services to organized groups of citizens, usually employee groups. These contracts supply physicians' services through health maintenance organizations (HMOs), either as closed groups or as independent practice associations (IPAs) through preferred provider organizations (PPOs) or as some variation of these two plans. In these settings, as we will see, the physician's autonomy is significantly diminished (see also Gurevitz 1984).

The HMO, which combines group practice with prepaid medical care, first appeared in 1929, although mental health services were not included until the late 1960s. Bennett (1988), in tracing the evolution of the HMO, emphasizes the change in purpose over the years, from idealism and collaboration to corporate profitability and competition, reflecting Ginzburg's (1984) "monetarization of medical care." Bennett notes the current trend toward IPAs, "open systems" of geographically dispersed mental health professionals, who engage in fee-for-service practice, as well as belonging to one or more HMOs. In 1984–1985, 71% of the 92 new HMOs were IPAs (Page 1987), and the trend may continue. Lacking the opportunities provided by HMOs of a closed group for education, development of a collegial culture, and incentives for innovation, IPAs are likely to diverge even more from the original goals of the HMO. Moreover, according to Bennett, since no internal group mechanisms exist to maintain cost effectiveness, IPAs rely on benefit constraints and retrospective utilization reviews, mechanisms that are apt to be intrusive and adversarial. Thus, Bennett says, "Control, rather than education, alliance, and collaboration, is the dominant theme" (p. 1547).

Bennett concludes that these changes in HMOs have introduced three major factors into the health delivery system: "1) an emphasis on the competitive ethic and on profit, 2) the professionalization of health care management, and 3) preoccupation with quantitative and technical dimensions of practice. Each has a profound impact on medical practice" (p. 1547).

The IPAs, PPOs, and HMOs of today will no doubt continue to expand or merge, moving, along with other industrial organizations, toward diversified, giant structures. These large organizations will provide fiscally effective but impersonally managed health care, wherein cost-benefit ratios and profitability become major determinants in the delivery of health care services. Already, 26.5% of the population seeking mental health care is serviced by such managed-care organizations (National Association of Private Psychiatric Hospitals 1988). Even governmental programs are now being contracted out to private health care programs, the most recent example being the CHAMPUS Reform Initiative (Zimet 1989).

The prevailing pressure to organize medical practice, including psychiatric and psychotherapeutic practice, into large multiservice corporations that competitively "sell" health care to the public on a large scale is a reflection of a more general trend in our economic system. The past decades have witnessed an unprecedented growth of multinational conglomerates that dominate a particular market. The automobile and oil industries are essentially divided among only a few companies. The same is becoming true of agriculture and travel services such as airlines. Whether this mode of manufacturing products is applicable to service industries remains debatable, the deterioration in the quality of air travel after "deregulation" being an instructive case in point.

Starr (1982) comments that, since the beginning of this century, large corporations have increasingly dominated all aspects of economic life. He contends that the small businessman or entrepreneur may be rooted in the American imagination but not in the American economy. The majority of the labor force now works for either government bureaucracies or private conglomerates; medical practitioners sooner or later had to conform to business trends toward bureaucratization.

Starr (1982) believes that the relative shortage of physicians and the increased cost of medical care are responsible for corporations and government gaining control of medical practice. While these factors were evoking bureaucratic expansion into health care delivery, the organization of public services was being largely transferred to private enterprise. Thus, instead of government managed national health insurance, the result has been corporate, for-profit regulation of medical care.

In regard to medical practice, proponents of this state of affairs argue simply that large organizations, corporate or governmental, can deliver services more efficiently than solo practitioners because of the economy of scale. Increasing reliance on expensive technical equipment and on standard laboratory tests for diagnosis and treatment is cited to support the view that medical practice has become a relatively predictable service with expectable costs and routine procedures. In this context, it is argued that extensive face-to-face contact between physician and patient has become progressively less central to many forms of medical care, as more diagnostic and treatment procedures are delegated to non-medical personnel. Whether this situation also applies to psychiatry, especially psychotherapy, which relies more on personal involvement than on applied technology for appropriate service, has not been considered in most health planning.

Centralized planning and regulation do produce tangible benefits to the consuming public. Psychiatrists, when left unregulated, have not satisfactorily allocated their resources in the best interests of the public. They have devoted much of their effort to caring for those patients who are "good" patients for treatment, rather than those who have the greatest need for treatment. Nevertheless, a distinction must be made between the corporate goal of profitability as determining health care delivery and the governmental goal of allocating a limited resource for the widest social benefit, even though both goals employ cost-containment methods. The federal administration in the 1980s tended to blur this distinction by applying corporate and business ethics to governmental endeavors, replacing the goal of satisfying social needs with one of bottom-line profitability. In some instances "privatization" of hitherto governmental activities was advocated.

The other major transformation of medical care resulting from general economic trends is the characterization of the patient as a consumer. Patients are seen as customers who will purchase competing health care packages, either directly or through their employers. Marketing and advertising campaigns present a variety of plans with varying degrees of misrepresentation, since, as Bennett (1988) points out, "in a competitive environment characterized by slick advertising and aggressive marketing, there is little likelihood that limitations will be emphasized" (p. 1547). The net result is that health care is viewed as a product to be sold on the open market and subject to the same pressures of cost effectiveness as a manufactured item. Again, we must question the appropriateness of this consumerist approach to the practice of psychiatry and psychotherapy, if not to all of medicine.

Ginzburg (1988) maintains that the for-profit sector of national medical expenditures has peaked and is likely to decline in the future. Whether explicitly for-profit health care organizations continue to grow or are replaced by other forms of managed health care, the fact remains that cost containment will have a continuing profound influence on health care delivery. The rise of a cadre of professional health care managers and the continuing dominance of third-party insurers will promote ongoing emphasis on cost effectiveness.

Present and future evidence that early mental health intervention ultimately benefits employers and society (Holden and Blose 1987: Mumford et al. 1984) may prove convincing to health care conglomerates and insurers, so that psychiatric services will play a continuing role in this system. However, the *nature* and *quality* of these services will probably be strictly determined and controlled largely by administrators who have had no psychiatric training. Thus mental health services may, in such systems, be limited to symptom relief and brief interventions, with emphasis on less expensive group therapy. (One of the few exceptions may be Medicare, which provides for unlimited outpatient psychotherapy.)

This trend has already provoked alarmed criticism. HMOs have been accused of selecting out high-risk patients by enrolling younger and healthier employees, while neglecting the older, more chronically ill patients, who then must be cared for by overburdened public facilities. The question of whether an HMO can care adequately for chronic illness at a competitive cost is repeatedly being raised. Senior citizens have complained to their Congressmen about the care they received at HMOs, provoking a move to enforce peer review on HMO practices (Evelyn 1987).

Another example of complaints about HMOs is found in a newspaper article (Dezell 1988). The story is told of a young woman, depressed over a recent miscarriage and work stress, who sought help from her HMO. She is quoted:

I waited what I felt was an inordinate amount of time to get an appointment. I asked to see a therapist in September and was given an appointment in late November. Then everything got put on hold because one worker was sick. So I went to *another* woman, and she laid this number on me about referring me to another waiting list to do group work. Well,

I wasn't interested in group work. I was in a crisis—crying
every day, in an extremely stressful job. I told her that, and
she started asking why I was so resistant to the notion of
group therapy. She told me that I really ought to examine
that. I had never sought therapy before, and I was getting hit
with one hurdle after another even though they knew I'd had
a miscarriage. Then to have this stuff laid on me as if it were
my own neurosis was just too much. (Dezell 1988, p. 4)

In the same article a benefits manager at "a major Bos-
ton-area high-tech company" is quoted: "The way HMOs
deal with staffing, with provider credentials, with waiting
time—the way they put up barriers to getting mental-health
care—sets up a process that does not allow for the delivery
of adequate, comprehensive health care" (Dezell 1988, p. 4).
Moreover, the director of the Harvard Community Health
Plan, a staff-model HMO, appears to reflect the policy of
many HMOs, when he is quoted in this article as saying, "We
don't believe long-term growth psychotherapy is within our
benefit. Our challenge has been to try to develop a short-term
approach to a broad population -- to take all comers and
develop short-term treatment programs for them. About 15
to 25 percent of our therapy is done in groups. We'd like to
see more" (p. 4).

There is no question but that brief therapy and group
therapy are effective modalities of treatment when they are
appropriately indicated by the patient's pathology. Yet it is
unlikely that in any other field of medicine one would find
such a Procrustean advocacy of a very limited treatment
range ("a short-term approach"), for "all comers," regardless
of diagnosis, solely on the basis of economic expediency.

Bennett (1988), in his discussion of the effects of managed care through HMOs in the mental health field, states

This concern [about mental health services cost] will create
pressure to exclude unprofitable patients, i.e., those with
major mental illness and disability, the aged, those at risk for
costly care, and those with the fewest active advocates. It will
militate against less quantifiable forms of treatment, such as
psychotherapy, by eliminating them, limiting access to them,

discouraging their use, or constructing benefits so that members pay separately for them. We are likely to witness allocation of professional time on the basis of ability to pay rather than need. Ironically, this reintroduces the problem of overtreatment of the few at the expense of the many, a situation that prompted the reform movement [of HMOs] in the first place. (p. 1548)

There will always be need for longer term, exploratory or supportive psychotherapeutic treatment for dysfunctional individuals and for the chronically mentally ill; however, such services, if offered at all in the managed-care context, will come under strict scrutiny and demands for their repeated justification. Utilization management, that is, the case-by-case assessment of services by an outside case manager prior to provision of those services, is on the rise. Now being implemented in traditional indemnity insurance plans, it is having a profound impact on hospital psychiatry; it will soon be extended to the outpatient side, as well.

A study of 205 HMOs found that over 80% offered the standard benefits of 20 outpatient visits or less (Levin and Glasser 1984). In one San Diego IPA, although 20 treatment sessions are covered by the insurance carrier, only 3 sessions are permitted without authorization. If further sessions are recommended by the provider, a report must be filed in order to obtain authorization for each 6 subsequent sessions. It is unusual for the full 20 sessions to be authorized, despite the fact that such coverage is advertised as being provided. Providers for another managed-care "gatekeeper" organization are told that their patterns of practice will be carefully monitored and that "overuse," regardless of what coverage is available to the patient, will result in their being dropped from the panel. CHAMPUS now requires reports every 10 sessions for further authorization of treatment. For a patient in twice-a-week exploratory therapy, continued treatment is in jeopardy every month—hardly a secure treatment environment in which to work out problems.

Not only will predetermined treatment formats probably be imposed upon patient/consumer and therapist alike even more widely than at present, but cost-effectiveness will determine the training backgrounds of mental health providers hired to offer services. It seems unlikely that psychiatrists will play a major role as psychotherapists in such organizations, except in doing brief, medication-assisted therapy. Rather they will provide psychopharmacological, supervisory, and administrative functions, as noted earlier.

It *does* seem likely that unregimented intensive psychotherapy and psychoanalysis will continue to be available in the next century of health care. This treatment, however, will generally be provided by psychotherapists *outside* the confines of the corporate health industry and third-party insurers. If managed health care continues on an impersonal and restrictive course, a significant number of patients will opt for private medical care to obtain more personalized treatment. A physician, who spent some time in a foreign country with government sponsored HMO services in which patients could enroll, found that many patients preferred to see their doctors privately (Noshpitz, personal communication, October 1989). Despite the HMO service being free after an initial fee, patients paid for care so as to have a continued relationship with a doctor whom they knew and trusted.

Individual practitioners and small group practices and clinics will remain but will probably represent a much smaller proportion of psychotherapists than today. They may well be viewed, even more than at present, as an "odd lot," a small contingent outside the mainstream of organized psychiatry, functioning as a professional "cottage industry," with its medical practitioners competing with less costly psychotherapists from different professional disciplines. Borus (1989) pointed out that the future market will be unable to support anywhere near the estimated 56% of psychiatrists in private practice in the mid-1980s (Fenton 1987).

Effects on the Patient

Perhaps the most significant effect of removing long-term exploratory psychotherapy from the roster of reimbursable treatments is the occurrence of treatment failures where long-term therapy is required but only psychopharmacological therapy or short-term therapies are available. It may be argued that this phenomenon is not new and that when economic factors prevent the application of an appropriate therapeutic modality, treatment failures have always occurred and certainly do occur today.

Frank acknowledgment of social injustice, that the world is not "fair," and that one may not be able to get what one wants or even needs, is a healthy recognition of reality and one that may promote therapeutic growth. However, in a society where the provision of all necessary health care by employers or other insurers is implied in coverage plans, social pressures may well tend to obscure this recognition. Already one sees the rationalizations for restricting coverage: that treatment is not "necessary" for "the worried well," that most, if not all, those who undergo long-term exploratory therapy are seeking "Cadillac frills," instead of "basic Ford" treatment. Currently in many settings, no outpatient psychotherapy of any duration whatsoever is provided, and care is limited to medication and crisis management.

Confronted with this kind of restricted care, patients may become convinced that their problems are only due to "chemical imbalance" and that drugs are the best that can be offered. When treatment failure occurs as a result of only partial treatment, the pervasive influence of such societally or institutionally encouraged beliefs will tend to make it more difficult for patients to face honestly the need either to settle for less-than-optimal results or to seek appropriate treatment outside the reimbursable mainstream. Patients may conclude that their problems cannot be treated, that personality or character cannot be changed.

As an example, members of a family sought help for neurotic difficulties at an HMO. Although their problems were eminently treatable with long-term psychotherapy, they were instead given antianxiety medication. They were told that "the rest is a matter of life style and emotions" and that they would "have to go home and work on that problem" themselves.

A response of that kind can evoke feelings of shame or guilt. The patient may come to feel that he or she is bad, defective, weak, ungrateful, and undeserving for failing to get well in the prescribed number of sessions. In other instances, a paranoid defense may be invoked, leading to the belief that the authorities, the bosses, etc., are deliberately keeping him or her downtrodden and in thrall by refusing to provide coverage.

A common covert transference reaction where third-party payers are involved, requiring careful attention, is the patient's (usually unconscious) fantasy that the therapist is personally responsible for limiting the treatment. This fantasy stems from the therapist's presumed participation in a relationship with the third-party payer (or supervisor), from which the patient feels painfully excluded, as a child feels excluded from the parental relationship. The patient may attempt to induce the therapist to join him or her in a rebellion against the "authoritarian" third party, especially if the patient senses the therapist feels guilty over conflict between loyalty toward the patient and loyalty to the HMO employer (J. Hoffman, personal communication, November 1988). A therapist who is particularly vulnerable may then collude with the patient to "get around the system," rather than helping the patient to consider ways of obtaining improved benefits.

This collusion may be particularly acute in those HMOs that permit continued treatment of certain patients, in "exceptional" instances. A two-track system may then develop, in which "special" patients who are the recipients of the therapist's positive countertransference receive longer treatment than other patients do. Patients who fit the therapist's idiosyncratic unconscious needs may be treated differently than those who, perhaps just as needy, are made to abide by the limitations set by the HMO.

In any event, if sufficient disability remains after the limit of treatment sessions is reached, provision will have to be made for alternative treatment. Presumably this will be at some community-supported mental health facility. For the most part, in these settings only supportive therapy of very limited frequency is available. Patients, already burdened by their reactions to treatment failure noted above, will tend to experience the referral as a humiliating confirmation of these fears. Patients with this iatrogenic syndrome may well require considerable work with a therapist to prevent a regressive retreat into permanent disability.

On the other hand, in many communities, individuals who otherwise would have been unable to obtain *any* psychotherapeutic treatment would get *some* treatment. The increased availability and probable wider utilization of psychiatric care should promote greater acceptance of psychiatric treatment as a nonstigmatized right. This acceptance, in turn, may encourage greater social efforts toward the provision of adequate treatment.

In a system of managed health care, the physician's performance is under periodic review. A further indirect advantage to patients will accrue from the resultant increased accountability and quality control. Any such system will tend to have a homogenizing effect on competence, constraining the best but ousting the worst. Such monitoring may be stifling and intimidating; however, there currently is *no* quality control for psychotherapists (or physicians, in general, who have an office-based practice) once their training is completed, except for limited peer review and whatever is occasioned by malpractice suits. Recognition of this problem has occasioned recurrent calls for periodic relicensure or recertification examinations.

Moreover, practice in a group setting makes it less likely that the patient will be forced into the favorite treatment modality of an individual therapist, regardless of its appropriateness. In addition, in the event of treatment failure, the patient is more likely to be referred for consultation to a colleague.

Effect on the Therapist

Each context for the practice of psychotherapy—ranging from the large, impersonal, industrial health care monolith to the small, isolated, entrepreneurial private practice—will have differing impacts on the psychotherapist. In addition, even though the setting for private psychotherapeutic practice may well be similar in the next century, it will have different meanings by virtue of its relation to the industrial health care organizations of that time.

The problems of adaptation that the future psychotherapist, working in the conglomerate health care system, will face are liable to be numerous. They will include: 1) problems of professional identity, at least for the medical practitioner; 2) ethical and moral problems generated specifically by the pressure to prescribe inadequate treatment; 3) frustrations arising from the frequent therapeutic failures resulting from externally imposed constraints; 4) the overestimation of therapeutic skills because the constraints on the duration of therapy protect against the recognition of personal therapeutic limitations; 5) personal doubts and problems for the psychotherapist who elects to practice outside of the mainstream (that is, the large health care structure); and 6) constriction of therapeutic experiences available for professional learning and development.

For many generations, students have chosen to study medicine, not only because of the wide scope of career options open to them as physicians but also because of the potential freedom to practice autonomously. This appeal has been similar for psychiatric physicians and, as private practice opportunities have increased, for nonphysician psychotherapists, as well. There has always been the option of affiliation with larger organizations, such as public treatment facilities, academic departments of psychiatry, or other health care programs. Although psychotherapy, when freed from fiscal constraints, can be effectively practiced in such settings, each of these alternatives to full-time psychotherapeutic practice has usually been selected because of other motives than a preference for seeing patients in such a setting. These motives may include wishes to teach, to do research, or to do administrative work.

If managed treatment facilities continue to proliferate and merge, most psychiatric treatment, especially brief, symptom-oriented psychotherapy, will be offered in such settings, and the autonomous, private practice setting will become progressively more anachronistic. The sharp curtailment of professional freedom and self-determination in the choice of length and depth of therapy will likely frustrate and alienate the psychotherapist who expects to make his or her own therapeutic decisions. Surrounded by colleagues who trivialize motivations to practice long-term, exploratory psychotherapy and who submit their therapeutic practice to fiscal and managerial criteria, the professional identity of those psychotherapists who are unable to practice their profession as they had hoped is likely to suffer.

Another stress on psychotherapists in the reimbursable mainstream, especially in an HMO, will be the pressure to prescribe and conduct a therapy that they may believe to be inadequate and inappropriate for certain patients. It is true that even in individual fee-for-practice medicine one must compromise with economic reality. Moreover, bureaucratic constraints that have to be coped with are nothing new. However, in the instance of psychotherapy, such conflicts take on an added dimension, especially in the context of transference phenomena. Not only are psychotherapists acting as treating professionals, but also, at least in the patient's mind, they are acting as representatives of the marketeer of the "health product" sold to patients as part of the employment "benefits" (and usually without their having had much choice in the matter).

What to tell the patient constitutes a dilemma. Simply to offer the inadequate therapy without making the therapist's opinions known to the patient is to be essentially dishonest by fostering false hopes for definitive resolution of the patient's problems. On the other hand, to inform the patient that the treatment about to be administered is probably going to be inadequate, but adequate treatment is not permitted by the HMO, is to compromise seriously any chance of success and to amplify manifold resistances.

Economic conflict of interest between patient needs and therapist needs certainly exists in private practice, as well. Private practitioners of psychotherapy are rarely so finan-

cially secure that they never experience the slightest temptation to see a patient at reduced frequency for their standard
fee, rather than reducing the fee or referring the patient to a
colleague who will accept a reduced fee, so that more adequate treatment may be obtained. Nor are private practitioners always free from the temptation to keep well-paying
patients in therapy longer than necessary if there are many
empty hours in their practices (the converse of the temptation
in managed care settings). Salaried practice in an organized
setting can eliminate this kind of conflict of interest and
source of financial anxiety for the psychotherapist.

The point is *not* whether conflict of interest also exists
in private practice. It does, but the private practitioner presumably struggles *against* the economic temptation, while
the HMO of today embraces and institutionalizes the economic solution to the conflict. One result in managed care
settings is the tendency to accept patient resistance to increased frequency or duration of therapy as reality and, in
consequence, to deny the reality of the patient's need.

Psychotherapy provided within managerial constraints will be successful only for those patients whose
problems fit into predetermined diagnostic molds, and an
increased number of therapeutic failures would inevitably
result. The impact of these additional failures will constitute
a further stress on the professional self-esteem of the practitioner. Conceivably, a negative feedback loop could result,
wherein reactions to increased therapeutic failures impair
subsequent therapeutic ability, ultimately leading to doubts
about therapeutic efficacy in general.

Therapists might well convince themselves that personality disorders are incurable, whatever treatment is provided, that psychoanalysis or exploratory psychotherapy is
futile for those who "really need" to alter their character, and
is only a form of self-indulgence for healthy individuals who
could function just as well without it. Thus assured that only
symptom reduction is possible, therapists would feel no
conflict about stopping treatment once the blatant clinical
manifestations of illness had subsided.

Conversely, therapeutic failures within restricted treatment confines might lead therapists to "walk away" from patients who failed to respond relatively quickly. They could then defensively deny their therapeutic limitations with the fantasy that, if only they had greater freedom to pursue treatment, all patients would ultimately improve under their ministrations. Thus, the limitations of psychotherapy or of one's own therapeutic capacities would never have to be confronted or experienced. As a consequence of working within constraints imposed by the health care system, this significant maturational task—so essential to development of therapist as well as patient—might in this way be evaded.

The psychotherapist working within a large health care system is unquestionably afforded significant advantages as well as disadvantages. The opportunity for easy consultation within a collegial group setting counteracts the professional isolation so characteristic of individual psychotherapeutic work and may promote a healthy bridging of theoretical differences.

J. Hoffman (personal communication, November 1988) has noted the following advantages: 1) the opportunity to work with a team; 2) regular and predictable working hours; 3) freedom from the business pressures of running a private practice; 4) seeing patients with a generally high degree of motivation; and 5) the opportunity to provide psychiatric consultation and liaison for primary care providers. Because the patients remain with the same group of physicians, the psychiatrist is able to maintain liaison more easily and monitor the psychiatric aspects of the long-term care being offered by the primary physicians.

The frustrations she describes are: 1) the common lack of provision of long-term exploratory psychotherapy, even for those patients for whom it is clearly indicated; 2) the common exclusion of significant groups of patients, such as chronic schizophrenic patients and patients with eating disorders; 3) limitations on the duration of inpatient treatment; and 4) insufficient psychiatric staffing, leading to psychiatrists finding their time heavily, or even exclusively, committed to medication management.

So far, we have examined the impact of a dominant managed health care delivery system on the medical or nonmedical psychotherapist working within this system. These issues may be sharpened by examining more specifically the challenges to that group of psychiatrists who will elect to leave the mainstream of managed health care delivery and operate in the "cottage industry" of private practice. These psychiatrists, aligned as they would be with similarly disposed psychologists, social workers, and other professionals, may risk confusion in their professional identity, reflected in conflicting allegiances both to psychotherapy and to medicine. This dilemma would resemble that of many psychoanalysts today, who worry about whether to pay dues and attend meetings only of their narrow psychoanalytic association or their broader psychiatric associations, or to do both.

Psychoanalytically oriented therapists (especially psychiatrists whose therapist-colleagues will, by and large, come from other disciplines) will understandably experience alienation from their medical colleagues, whose practice will be perceived as different. As they compare themselves to their peers, this sense of difference may elicit feelings of shame and doubt (Morrison 1989) or, conversely, feelings of superiority. In the past, psychoanalysts experienced themselves with pride as being at the prestigious, cutting edge of the profession. However, in the future they might have to deal with feelings of isolation from peers, perhaps accompanied by a sense of shame or guilt over being out of the mainstream. These physicians may forge new alliances with nonphysicians, but at the cost, perhaps, of further exclusion and ridicule by the bulk of medically and pragmatically oriented psychiatrists, evoking further doubts and shame. Such feelings add to the "burnout" phenomenon for analytically oriented psychiatrists practicing in solo contexts, already committed to a craft that itself leads to isolation from peers and institutions. The absence of support, direction, and collegial exchange that might be provided in managed health care settings would accentuate self-doubts, and the resultant stress and challenges to self-esteem might well cause many

private practitioners to turn from their depth-psychothera-
peutic practices to other endeavors (including, for many,
joining the health care establishment).

The psychotherapist who elects to operate outside of the
system, practicing according to conviction, faces not only a
degree of professional isolation, but also limitations on refer-
rals and remuneration. Of course, such conditions recreate
many of the circumstances practitioners formerly faced
when psychodynamic psychiatry was born. These circumstances could lead (and may have led then) to a sense of
defiance which might have significant countertransference
repercussions. For example, in the treatment of adolescents
caught up in autonomy struggles with controlling parents,
the therapist might identify with and support elements of the
struggle that would seem quite different, were the therapist
not involved in similar confrontations with the health care
system. These countertransference elements would of necessity become part of the self-examination required for the
practice of open-ended treatment.

Pressures for respectability, as well as for reimbursement, will often conflict with professional convictions about
what is appropriate treatment. Practitioners will often have
to compromise their activities in order to receive payment.
Progressively more stringent constraints on practice will be
imposed through peer review and official treatment guidelines. Ultimately, these constraints may result in legal pressures to comply with dominant treatment criteria. Imposed
from without, they would confront the therapist with the
need to act against deeply held beliefs and ideals.

The foregoing is not to be construed as a criticism of peer
review. It is one valid way to deal with the sometimes conflicting goals of cost containment and quality control and also
serves as a helpful educational process for the practitioner.
Since 1978, the American Psychiatric Association has published a Peer Review Manual, which has always included
criteria for the prescription and concurrent review of psychoanalysis, as well as criteria for exploratory, symptom-relief
oriented, supportive, and focal psychotherapies. However,
the assumption made in peer-review activities is that quality

control will effect cost containment by reducing waste and ineffective treatment, not by eliminating necessary modalities of treatment (as in managed health care) just because they may be less profitable.

On a more practical level, insurance premiums for malpractice may rise significantly, depending on how much psychotherapeutic practice deviates from established norms. This rise in premiums will bring to bear yet another influence on how the solo practice of psychotherapy is conducted. An added element of fear would be a further burden on the solo psychotherapist and contribute to the countertransference. On the face of it, these problems of alienation for the private practitioner of psychotherapy seem ominous and discouraging. On the other hand, a movement toward a separate "cottage industry" may paradoxically afford the possibility for rejuvenation. In banding together as a dedicated, beleaguered minority, psychoanalytically oriented psychotherapists might recapture the pioneering spirit and energy that once infused their practice.

Effect on Education

In the previous section, we considered the ways in which the practice of psychotherapy might become influenced by its incorporation into a widespread managed health care system. The nature of psychotherapy *training* would also inevitably be influenced, especially in traditional medical settings, such as medical schools and residency training. Psychotherapy would increasingly be viewed in the context of the managed health care setting, and those techniques that fit well in such settings—short-term, group, symptomatic relief, and supportive therapies—would be emphasized and preferred. Far more attention in residency programs would be given to training in group psychotherapy, brief symptom relief, or focal therapy, compared to long-term modalities. If conglomerates continue to integrate with and even buy out centers of medical training (as has already occurred in some areas), this influence on psychotherapy education will become increasingly more widespread.

As current constraints continue progressively to limit the numbers and types of patients that are treated in open-ended psychotherapy, many important factors that have shaped the training and experience of therapists and psychoanalysts will be lost. For example, if trainees have limited access to long-term exploratory work with angry, primitively organized patients, they will not have the experience of dealing with chronic, unremitting negative transferences. Although in some ways this absence might be considered a relief, it would also deny the developing therapist the resistant anvil against which to forge and shape clinical skills that are equally useful in short term therapy and psychopharmacological management. Once the going got rough, beginning therapists, never having experience with the gradual resolution of transference attitudes, would be inclined to give up too soon.

Similarly, limited experience with such angry patients would deprive the therapist of the experience of the gradual, long-term process of working through such resistant, early problems as distrust and projected rage, within the transference and countertransference. In general, the lack of experience in observing long-term changes in patients will deprive the student psychiatrist of the vital dimension of understanding the long-term forces that shape human lives for better or for worse—again, an understanding that is extremely valuable in the application of other modalities of psychiatric treatment.

Within the unconstrained, open context of long-term exploratory work, with its regressive transference vicissitudes, therapist and patient alike learn to tolerate the inevitable ambiguities of therapy (as of life itself). When the treatment is predetermined by length, outcome criteria, or oversight, both parties are denied access to the uncertainties of both process and outcome, which, in fact, may be one of the essentials in the process of personal restoration offered by this form of treatment. Experiential knowledge of the vagaries of a long-term therapeutic relationship and its transferences—an essential element of therapeutic ambiguity (Adler 1989)—would be curtailed by the pressures of cost containment. The inevitable shifts in valence and dynamic equilibrium of such a long-term relationship would be un-known—to therapist and patient alike—and both would thus be denied an opportunity to generalize such shifts from the therapeutic transference to other relationships. Exter-nally imposed constraints could lead to a distorted belief that the therapeutic relationship, and, by extension, other affec-tionate ties, must always be exact, clear from the beginning, and quick to resolve.

Again, we do not intend to imply that briefer kinds of therapy are not as valuable as long term therapy. Given the appropriate indications (Offenkrantz et al. 1982), focal ther-apy is a most effective modality of treatment; and in a previ-ous publication we have documented its efficacious use (GAP Committee on Therapy 1978). Were *it* in danger of being abolished, we would as vigorously argue against such a loss.

Another possible consequence of the lack of long-term exploratory therapy training is the insufficient development of a capacity to arrive at a psychodynamic formulation. Such a formulation stresses an evaluation not only of the precipi-tating events in the patient's life but their interaction with the patient's past vulnerabilities and defenses and often requires several interviews to develop fully. It allows the clinician to decide on a therapeutic approach in work with the patient and to anticipate the difficulties that can arise in the treat-ment, including transference and countertransference prob-lems.

The failure to learn and apply such skills has an impact that goes well beyond the ability to conduct individual long-term psychotherapy. For example, a patient was admitted to a short-term inpatient unit by his behaviorally oriented ther-apist for psychopharmacological treatment of his obsessive-compulsive disorder and major affective disorder. He rap-idly provoked the staff into believing that he had neither disorder but was merely "manipulative" and therefore should be discharged. Neither the inpatient unit nor the therapist had done a psychodynamic evaluation. Had they done so, it would have defined this patient's long-term character problems, with his self-defeating behavior and repeated use of projective identification, which had become re-enacted with the therapist and hospital. A proper formulation that understood these factors could have worked out a behavioral strategy that addressed the longer term personality problems. Proper attention would have been given to the transference and countertransference implications, avoiding the impasse and resultant hospital discharge that were destructive to this patient.

As we have noted, training and education in long-term exploratory psychotherapy and psychoanalysis will no doubt continue to some extent. However, such training is likely to be conducted in specialized, multidisciplinary institutes and training centers, far removed from the usual contexts of medical training. On the other hand, there is evidence, particularly in the Northeast United States, that such freestanding centers may themselves become integrated with the larger medical training institutions, primarily for economic reasons. Such integration could generate another source of teachers of long-term exploratory psychotherapy to psychiatric residents in academic training centers, but will not begin to approach the need for teachers in remoter sections of the country.

We have noted the shift away from emphasis on psychoanalysis and long-term exploratory psychotherapy, which dominated the interest and investment of most psychiatric training centers for residents and medical students from the 1940s until the mid-1960s. Competition for attention and teaching time came from psychopharmacology, starting in the late 1950s, from community psychiatry in the 1960s, and recently from biological psychiatry. Many suggest that long-term exploratory psychotherapy is losing the competition, while others believe that it is retreating from an overinflated position to a more realistic place along with these other subdisciplines of psychiatry. It is perhaps significant that, concomitant with the declining emphasis in the teaching of psychotherapy in residency training programs, increasing numbers of freestanding psychoanalytic training centers are mounting psychotherapy training programs in addition to their psychoanalytic training curricula.

Currently, private practitioners of psychoanalytic psychotherapy still serve an important function in many departments of psychiatry, both as supervisors of psychodynamic diagnostic and psychotherapeutic skills for psychiatric residents (Offenkrantz et al. 1982) and as teachers of dynamic psychiatry to medical students. However, if this role and those skills become detached from core psychiatric teaching, the solo practitioner will find increasingly limited space in medical education. Where once these individuals served as the major role models (frequently as chairmen) in psychiatric departments, they will become progressively more remote from psychiatric education. Instead, they will continue to teach in multidisciplinary programs and institutes devoted to the transmission of psychotherapeutic skills, functioning outside of the mainstream centers for psychiatric training. This alienation from medical teaching will lead to further isolation of the psychotherapist from psychiatry.

In a previous GAP report by the Committee on Therapy (1986), arguments were advanced for the purely educational value to the psychiatrist of learning long-term exploratory psychotherapy. These arguments will be as valid in the future as they are today. There is no better way to study aspects of human experience, such as transference, fantasy function and formation, dreams, and the so-called psychopathology of everyday life—aspects which will continue to inform psychiatric practice. Moreover, the attitudinal skills generated by experience and supervision in this kind of psychotherapy are essential to the optimum functioning of the psychiatrist in all areas of practice. For such supervision to continue, however, appropriate cases must continue to be made available for this treatment.

Trainees in more rural or smaller programs may have no actual experience at all in long-term psychotherapy during their residency years. Such a deficiency will lead to a large number of graduate psychiatrists who lack this skill. Chances are that this group of new practitioners, being unable to deliver this service, will tend to denigrate the usefulness of not only long-term psychotherapy but possibly even of psychodynamic psychiatry in its entirety.

One interesting area of support for training in long-term exploratory psychotherapy may come from biological psychiatry itself. The studies of Eric Kandel (1989) and others demonstrate that learning (as in psychotherapy) demonstrably affects the brain, its structure, and its composition. In the not-so-distant future, the neurochemical, neuropsychological, and neuroanatomical correlates of long-term exploratory psychotherapy may be a major area of investigation and teaching. Teachers will be required who are conversant both in the neurosciences and in the psychodynamic underpinnings of long-term exploratory psychotherapy. Biological correlates of psychological ideas and psychological correlates of biological findings will help — far more than an outmoded metapsychology—to fulfill Freud's original goal of integrating biological and psychological constructs and firmly establish the scientific credibility of long-term exploratory psychotherapy (Kandel 1989).

The integration of psychoanalytic training centers into universities would favor the "rescue" of psychology by biology and provide psychoanalytic educators who are comfortable with the integration of brain and psyche. Should changes in the brain resulting from long-term exploratory psychotherapy be demonstrated, insurance companies and health care enterprises may have to take notice and begin to support these endeavors. In fact, it is biology that may ultimately assure that long-term exploratory psychotherapy is *not* relegated to the category of cottage industry.

Who, then, would be the teachers of the principles and practice of long-term exploratory psychotherapy and psychoanalysis? Clearly, one source would be those full-time academics who are fully trained in both psychoanalysis and biological psychiatry and who can comfortably integrate these two areas of psychiatric knowledge. Unfortunately, such people are rare in current departments of psychiatry. Currently one finds only an occasional resident or recent graduate working in a laboratory while pursuing some training in long-term psychotherapy. Were their numbers to increase, they would evoke a welcome countertrend in the field.

In the halcyon days of psychoanalysis, the most revered teachers of long-term exploratory psychotherapy were private practitioners identified more with psychoanalytic institutes than with academic departments of psychiatry. They taught several hours per week, often in their private offices. Currently, fewer heroes and ideological demigods exist as role models standing against the inevitable ambiguities of psychiatry, but there are more academics capable of balanced views and of integrating the complex universes of knowledge in our field.

A word of caution about the somewhat optimistic scenario outlined above. The future scientific demonstration, a la Kandel, of the *mechanism* of long-term exploratory psychotherapy would not necessarily demonstrate its *efficacy*. Moreover, even were efficacy demonstrated, this in itself would not ensure the inclusion of long-term exploratory psychotherapy in a health care system. At present, there are demonstrably effective medical procedures that are not reimbursable, and, conversely, many reimbursable procedures have not been demonstrated to be efficacious. Decisions as to inclusion of treatments in a health care program are primarily political and socioeconomic ones, with scientific proof of effectiveness only one factor to be considered.

Chapter 3

What Will the Service Be?

The outcome of the trend toward increasingly stringent limitations on both the duration and frequency of reimbursable psychotherapy seems clear. Long-term exploratory psychotherapy will become increasingly restricted to a relatively minuscule number of affluent patients who not only can afford to pay for such treatment but are also willing to do so outside of their health insurance plans. In an environment where almost all physicians will probably practice in prepaid health groups, the effect will be an essential removal of this modality of therapy from the armamentarium of the vast majority of practicing psychiatrists. The implications are likely to be manifold and far-reaching.

Psychotherapy will become, for the most part, limited to such briefer and time-limited modalities as symptom-relief, focal, and brief supportive therapies. In keeping with the techniques of these therapies, the roles of identification or introjection in promoting therapeutic results may play a larger role than that of insight. Differing opinions are expressed in the literature on focal therapy about what the appropriate focus of the treatment should be (for example, transference themes or oedipal themes, etc). Increased interest and study in the future may provide more standard procedures for this modality. Similarly, supportive therapy is likely to receive more study with the development of more clearly defined interventions.

Other forms of treatment will probably be combined
with individual psychotherapy: group therapy, behavior
modification, pharmacotherapy, and family therapy. Individual psychotherapy will increasingly assume the position
of an adjunct to these other forms of treatment. The focus of
the work will be narrowed to precipitating stresses and acute
exacerbations that may be treated within the reimbursable
framework. The always-important question in diagnostic
evaluations—"Why have you come at this particular time for
treatment"—will become even more crucial in planning interventions.

It is unlikely that exploratory psychotherapy of psycho-
ses will survive as a reimbursable endeavor, even as an
ancillary treatment. Perhaps minimal supportive contact
with the schizophrenic patient will be maintained in order to
obtain compliance with medication prescriptions. Similarly,
the long-term therapy of borderline personality disorder is
unlikely to be conducted, except as repeated crisis intervention to forestall hospitalization.

As an adaptation to the financial exigencies of insurance
plans, a variant of brief focal psychotherapy may well be
developed, namely *episodic psychotherapy*. Psychotherapy
will be conducted until treatment benefits are used up, then
discontinued with a plan to resume when a new fiscal period
starts. Such an approach carries with it inevitable problems
of disruption and loss of continuity of the therapy. Yet,
episodic periods of treatment may allow for a brief emphasis
on a particular problem, which can then be "practiced" by
the patient during the therapy-free period and reviewed
when therapy resumes, with an assessment of the growth
and mastery attained during the independent work. In some
instances, a new focus will have emerged, which can then be
explored during a new episode of treatment. The impact of
such a modality on patients with primary problems of sepa-
ration will probably be significant but remains to be explored.

Another possible adaptation to such fiscal reality may
be reflected in our diagnostic nomenclature and conceptions.
If no reimbursable treatment is available for an emotional

illness, such as a severe personality disorder, it is likely that the diagnosis will seldom, if ever, be used, and another will be substituted. Even now, diagnoses are made with an eye toward what is reimbursable. Thus psychopathology will become redefined in order to conform to the treatment methods that will be offered or reimbursed, with emphasis on those symptoms that are treatable by short-term psychotherapy with or without medication. Moreover, under a Resource-Based Value System (which will become the arbiter of fee scales in mental health care, as well as medicine in general) there will be incentives to make the most heavily reimbursable diagnosis. A similar phenomenon is occurring in hospital care, now under the sway of diagnosis-related groups (DRGs). Some physicians are complaining of subtle pressure by hospital administrators to give the patient a diagnosis that carries with it the greatest reimbursement. If, for example, a patient's psychotherapy is reimbursed at a higher rate if he or she is considered a suicidal risk (a proposal that is now under consideration), the incidence of reported suicidal risk may well show a significant rise. The danger of resultant stigmatization of the patient is a serious one.

Increasing attention and research will be devoted not only to more effective pharmacologic interventions, but also to ways in which the therapeutic results obtainable by long-term exploratory psychotherapy can be achieved with less frequent and shorter treatment periods. A substitute inducer of therapeutic intensity (or therapeutic regression), now enhanced by frequency of sessions, will be sought, perhaps with renewed interest in hypnotic or psychedelic states. Similarly, facilitators of learning will be investigated, in order to shorten the duration of treatment now required for certain characterologic changes. Perhaps innovative combinations of behavior modification with dynamic psychotherapy will be developed, in which the behavior modification is keyed not to the manifest symptomatic behavior, but to the unconscious dynamics underlying the symptoms, as understood by dynamically informed therapists. Changes will also occur in what is considered to constitute malpractice. Suits have

already been brought for using psychotherapy alone in depression and failing to prescribe an antidepressant. Perhaps
a future cause of legal action will be the allegation of unnec-
essary prolongation of psychotherapy.

Chapter 4

PROPOSALS

General Socioeconomic Issues

The purpose of this report has been to extrapolate trends created by the impact of changing socioeconomic realities on the practice of psychotherapy and to highlight possible future problems. While the problems may be readily identified, workable solutions are not so apparent. The application of a business ethos to an ostensibly humanitarian vocation is generating repercussions at many levels of society. Solutions of a general nature may be sought by changing major areas of society, or else by changing more specific aspects that pertain only to psychiatry.

Increasing Public Awareness

The marked transformation in health delivery that we have described has transpired with remarkably little concern or alarm expressed by patients/consumers, governmental agencies, or practicing physicians. Much of the public seems virtually unaware of the tremendous changes that are occurring in a most important sector of their welfare.

A few decades ago, there was a great deal of public debate and apprehension over the "danger" of national health insurance, which was seen as a forerunner of "creeping socialism" that would supposedly destroy our way of life.

At that time, the medical profession, with the aid of government and private groups, set up effective barricades to the
introduction of "socialized medicine." Now, in amazing contrast, entrepreneurial, for-profit health plans have perme-
ated a good deal of medical care without a whimper of
protest. Skillful marketing has presented these programs as
good for industry and patients (who would pay less for
health care), as well as good for physicians (who would have
more jobs and spend less time on nonmedical, business
aspects of practice). However, when the details (or realities)
of such programs have been scrutinized, the resultant picture
has not been so positive. Therefore, one overall approach to
coping with the inroads of corporate practices into health
care delivery is to increase both professional and public
awareness of what the realities of such a radical alteration
actually entail.

The need to inform the public is not only a matter of
physicians' self-interest (which should be freely acknowledged), but also may be considered an ethical obligation. A
nationwide sociomedical experiment is being performed,
and full disclosure of the risks must be made to the partici-
pants (Michels and Eth 1986). An educational campaign,
regarding the true mental health needs of any population,
should be aimed at both the public (that is, the consumers)
and at legislators on all levels of government. Such an effort
might result in more appropriate benefit packages. The data
showing such needs are already known in some detail, having been compiled by a number of epidemiologic studies
over the past 30 to 40 years (Barrett and Rose 1986; Robins et
al. 1984; Srole et al. 1962). The findings of such studies should
be brought to the attention of relevant parties, particularly
because the findings reveal such a high rate of dysfunction
secondary to mental illness.

There appears to be widespread denial by the public of
the extent of psychiatric impairment in our population, possibly because we wish to think of ourselves as sane, happy,
effective individuals. We do not want to hear facts that belie
an idealized self-concept. This same avoidance of painful
truths permitted alarming rates of child physical and sexual

abuse to continue unnoticed, until reporting of such activity became mandated by law.

This desire to see society, and ourselves, as mentally healthy works against obtaining adequate mental health ben efits from managed care systems and adequate protection from governmental agencies. Prospective clients may not scrutinize or evaluate mental health benefits offered by various programs, because they do not want to think of themselves as ever needing psychiatric care. Publicizing the real prevalence of mental illness and actual rates of disability secondary to psychiatric problems may encourage future enrollees in managed care systems—and their legislators—to insist on more extensive coverage.

There is a good possibility that, if these figures were called to the attention of industry, personnel departments would be less ready to agree to contract for comprehensive health services without mental health components. There are already signs that big business is having second thoughts about the ability of HMOs to fulfill the health needs of employees. Illinois Bell's director of benefits was quoted to the effect that fee-for-service insurance is superior to HMO coverage for alcoholism treatment and psychiatric care. One Minneapolis-based computer firm, which pioneered acceptance of HMOs, dropped such contracts in 1988 in favor of fee-for-service insurance (Evelyn 1987).

Many of the problems stemming from managed care that face psychiatry seem to be shared by most, if not all, medical practitioners. It is ironic that the same medical establishment, which was able to rally itself against the creation of a national health insurance program on the grounds that such a program would remove the control of medical practice from medical practitioners, has allowed private entrepreneurs to accomplish the realization of this most dreaded threat.

As the wheel turns full circle, a number of respected physicians are now speaking out in favor of a national health insurance program as the only solution to our nation's health woes (Einthoven and Kronick 1989). Moreover, business and labor are both evincing increased interest in such proposals.

There are now 37 million people in our country without any form of health insurance (Time Magazine 1990). If properly funded and managed, a national health insurance plan could provide an optimal structure wherein both short-term and long-term intensive psychotherapy could be provided to patients, according to need.

In a previous publication, we demonstrated the financial feasibility of including long-term psychotherapy in such a national health insurance plan, where the problems of adverse selection would not be encountered (GAP Committee on Therapy 1978). In other countries, including West Germany and Canada, even psychoanalysis has been successfully covered (at least to a considerable extent) for many years under a national health insurance plan.

Patient Protection and Advocacy

To explore the possibility of "large scale" solutions, some recognition must be given to a definite change in public mores. The doctor-patient relationship, formerly paternalistic with at least some elements of collegiality, has changed to one that is primarily contractual. This transformation is in keeping with a more general metamorphosis in American culture.

In *Habits of the Heart* by Bellah et al. (1986), a comprehensive examination of our current culture, the authors conclude that America has lost a sense of community, leaving individuals largely alienated from each other and lacking a feeling of trust or mutual commitment. Not so long ago, patients trusted their doctors, just as they trusted their grocers, repairmen, bankers, and so on. Individuals encountered in business transactions were known to one's family and community for years and had to give an honest account of themselves or lose their standing in a shared society. These individuals were also encountered outside of professional interchanges, as they shared one's communal universe and commitment to similar goals. The authors found that this collegial form of interpersonal relationships has all but disappeared. In its place is a uniform yet faceless array of products, be these in canned goods, TV programs, or health care. Psychiatry, as part of society, may be reflecting society's movement to a particular anomic phase of its history.

In such times of general alienation and amoral competitiveness in the marketplace, governmental regulation may be required to provide the protection to the consumer that previously had been guaranteed by familiarity or good will. Toward this end, a regulatory agency might be constituted to set standards and regulate HMOs and other health care delivery systems, just as the Food and Drug Administration monitors the marketing of possibly dangerous drugs or the Federal Aviation Administration oversees the safety of air travel. Such a watchdog agency might swell an already bursting bureaucracy and make organized medicine less attractive to the corporate world, but it would protect the rights of patients.

Even if such a governmental agency is not created, groups of patients and their families might form organizations whose task is to promote better care through political action. The National Alliance for the Mentally Ill (NAMI) has been formed to improve treatment received by chronic patients from public (and other) institutions. This nationwide organization perceives itself as a strong force for patient advocacy, with educative, political, and, most recently, research funding responsibilities. Other groups of patients (and their families) who receive less than optimal care could follow NAMI's example and seek to influence the allocation of psychiatric services.

Another kind of patient group that is gaining popularity and acquiring political influence is the self-help association, such as Alcoholics Anonymous. Victims of family violence, pathological gambling, substance abuse, and eating disorders are meeting with other afflicted individuals on their own initiative and are thus finding help outside the medical and mental health system. Other groups of patients, such as those with major affective disorder, are forming self-help groups to address their emotional and psychological needs that are not met by the medication obtained from their doctors. Although members of these groups receive medical care for the major symptoms of their illnesses, they rely on fellow patients for support and education in learning to cope with a lifelong illness. It is possible that groups like these may significantly supplement the role of traditional psychotherapy as a source of emotional support and interpersonal care. Since such groups cannot substitute for definitive psychotherapeutic care, where it is indicated, we hope that they will be sophisticated enough to support such definitive treatment.

Thus it is conceivable that in times of social estrangement, individuals who feel a lack of response to their needs on the part of government or the medical establishment will form their own networks of support systems based on shared concerns. These groups may use social action to obtain care or begin supplying it themselves.

Adaptation of Psychotherapy to Managed Care

There is a good possibility that, given the current trend, most of the healing professions will become part of managed care systems, despite the efforts noted above to forestall this change. The question to be addressed, then, is how modifications can be achieved that will allow more relevant delivery of psychotherapeutic services. In this connection, the American Psychiatric Association has established an Ad Hoc Committee on Managed Care. Its purpose is to explore ways to engage the managed care phenomenon in a manner helpful to both APA members and the patients they serve. The following are our specific proposals, which could be adapted to managed care systems without radically altering their basic philosophy.

A major salutary step would be a variable prescription of outpatient treatment for different psychiatric conditions. Coverage for all other fields of medicine is based on specific diseases rather than an arbitrary allotment of a set amount of time or expertise per year for any form of morbidity. Similarly, secondary, complicating factors that could influence recovery are taken into account. This form of flexible coverage, dependent on the type of psychiatric disorder, would help in providing appropriate care. A previous GAP report (GAP Committee on Therapy 1978), clearly indicated the differential requirements of psychotherapy for various disorders. It would be the task of psychotherapists to agree on optimal forms and durations of therapy with respect to diagnosis and complicating factors. Since appropriate forms of therapy would be covered, there would be less pressure to misdiagnose to obtain reimbursement, and peer review would then be able to control any such tendency.

In the idealistic origins of HMOs (see Bennett 1988), preventive services were clearly visualized. Some HMOs currently offer some such services, such as bereavement counseling that subscribers can request after a death in their family. These interventions have been of significant value but are always at risk of being sacrificed to cost containment. It will be imperative that "watchdog" functions exist within the managed health care system to prevent the loss of such creative approaches.

An even more formidable task is persuading managed care systems to agree to cover long-term exploratory forms of therapy. However, if it can be shown that such forms of therapy are actually cost-effective in the long run, such an agreement might be negotiated. HMOs and PPOs might also respect results that demonstrate that psychotherapy reduces the utilization of other medical facilities and may prevent future psychiatric hospitalization. Such data would explicitly support the contention that psychotherapy does result in significant life changes and that psychotherapy is most effective when conducted by experienced and adequately trained therapists.

The policy of variable lengths of treatment for specific individuals is already instituted in some HMOs, but in a manner that is both unofficial and unfair to the patient. In these cases, the patient is allowed a certain number of prepaid therapy visits per year. If the patient and the therapist agree that more visits are necessary (for example, more than

10 per year), the patient can continue but must pay an additional fee per visit. The fee is collected by the HMO, but the therapist is not given "caseload" credit for the additional therapy. On the one hand, the therapist is discouraged from exceeding the 10 visits, since additional visits increase his or her workload without recompense, even though the patient is paying for this service. On the other, this procedure represents a tacit admission that 10 (or whatever number) visits is arbitrary and not appropriate for the whole range of illnesses. It reveals the need for a variable schedule of therapy based on optimal response.

An alternative would be for insurers to develop graduated insurance packages, wherein coverage for outpatient psychotherapy ranged from a bare minimum of, say, 10 visits per year to one that covered 150 outpatient visits yearly for 3 years. The problem of adverse selection of the more liberal programs might be handled by requiring a very large co-payment, such as 70%, for the *first* 50 visits with a decreasing co-payment thereafter; or one could require a long waiting period of, say, 3 years before becoming eligible for the extended benefits. Although high co-payments and long waiting periods are traditionally considered to benefit the wealthy at the expense of the poor utilizers, this would not be true if alternative packages were available that had lesser coverage but low copayments.

Finally, psychiatric practice may have to be modified in order to reduce cost while hoping to supply adequate care. Schneider-Braus (1987) has outlined just such a set of proposed guidelines, arising from her experience as a psychiatrist working in an HMO. For her, effective treatment within an HMO setting requires the following. 1) A thorough intake evaluation must be done to facilitate triage for specific treatments. 2) The patient's real requests must be identified, with a concern for addressing conscious, verbalized needs. 3) A goal-oriented contract should then be negotiated by patient and therapist, with explanation of the limitations of the coverage to counteract later feelings of abandonment or disappointment. 4) The emphasis should be on symptom relief via focal therapy and specialty clinics. 5) Less costly treatments (such as group therapy and bibliotherapy) should be used, including the utilization of community supports (such as Alcoholics Anonymous). 6) An ego-enhancing, problem-solving attitude should be established with the patient, centering on current reality concerns and including discussion of economic limitations to promote therapeutic goals of limit setting, reality testing, and impulse control. (How impulse control is thus promoted is unclear.) 7) Termination should be facilitated after symptom relief. Schneider-Braus also recommends learning to work with the HMO review board in terms of how to appeal cases requiring more extensive treatment, and she emphasizes the need to conduct research to help determine future HMO policies.

Her article is as instructive for what it does not say, as it is for what it discusses. There is little space allotted for "consumer" disenchantment or anger, although the prospective HMO psychiatrist is advised to go over the "fine print" at the initial session. One senses that the patient is often unaware of the HMO's limitations on mental health coverage. There is no mention of how many patients are considered satisfactorily treated within the coverage limitations. The recommendations appear to preclude long-term insight directed therapy or any therapy not primarily oriented toward "problem solving" and "reality testing." Finally, the recommendations reveal how issues of the cost and extent of treatment seem to pervade the therapy, as if the patient and therapist have one eye on the cash register and the other on the clock.

J. Hoffman (personal communication, November 1988), from her experience as chief psychiatrist in an HMO, also recommends that there be maximum flexibility of the treatment team leader (preferably a psychiatrist). It is essential that he or she be familiar with all recognized treatment approaches for mental health problems. The same point is made by Bennett (1988), based on his experience at The Harvard Community Health Plan. Modifications toward a more realistic and humane approach to psychotherapy in managed care systems may evolve, as other therapists candidly report their professional experience in such settings, stating their gratifications and frustrations, as well as their educated recommendations.

Outcome and Efficacy Research

We strongly recommend that priority be given to continued research into the effectiveness of long-term exploratory psychotherapy, as complex and difficult as that research is. An increasing number of studies (GAP 1978; Kantrowitz et al. 1986, 1987; Luborsky et al. 1988) clearly demonstrate the beneficial effect of long-term exploratory therapy on relationships, on the ability to handle emotions, and on general health issues. Studies in West Germany, where psychoanalysis is covered under national insurance, have suggested its cost effectiveness in reducing general medical expenses in those patients who were so treated.

However, when limited health dollars must be allocated, explicit efficacy studies assume increasing importance and must be pursued. Equally important are adverse outcome data, so that we know more definitely when long-term exploratory therapy is *contraindicated*. Appreciation of the importance of such studies in medicine in general is reflected in the creation in January 1990, of the Federal Agency for Health Care Policy and Research with a multimillion dollar budget, which will be mandated to study "outcomes." Mindful of this need for research, the American Psychoanalytic Association has established a task force to explore how such research may be furthered.

Outcome and efficacy studies for less intensive long-term therapy are also needed. For example, it is believed by many that even once-weekly outpatient therapy in many instances forestalls hospitalization in borderline and other personality disorders, and may also reduce the recurrence of depression (Frank et al. 1989; Miller et al. 1989). Corporations that contract for health coverage for their employees would be impressed by figures demonstrating that absenteeism or disability, particularly secondary to substance abuse or psychosomatic illness, is reduced as a consequence of psychotherapy. At least one company, McDonnell Douglas, has found that provision of quality mental health care through Employee Assistance Programs (EAPs), though more expensive initially, saves millions of dollars yearly in excess medical costs (Winslow 1989). There is also a need for comparative outcome studies comparing the outcome of four- or five-times weekly psychoanalysis with twice-a-week long-term psychotherapy to determine explicitly which clinical constellations require the more intensive setting and which can be treated just as successfully with less intensive long-term methods.

Research could also assess both the cost effectiveness and the improved quality of life that may be achieved with selected borderline and chronic schizophrenic patients who are treated with once-weekly long-term psychotherapy. Such therapy is often described as "supportive" or "case management"; yet, as Wallerstein (1986) has found, even the most exploratory therapies have significantly more supportive elements than had been previously acknowledged, so distinctions of this kind are less useful. Research should be able to reveal whether 1) significant changes can occur, albeit slowly, in such work with these patients, and 2) whether these patients are also capable of benefitting from a degree of exploratory psychotherapy in a treatment that has many supportive elements.

In this era of short-term hospital stays for psychiatric illness, we believe that long-term inpatient psychotherapy is still indicated for certain patients, especially among those who have had previous hospital admissions or treatment failures in other settings. Yet research is needed to develop more explicit criteria for determining who will benefit from this treatment. Similarly definitive studies are needed on the benefits of inpatient treatment versus outpatient treatment for alcoholism.

Clinical outcome studies should be undertaken, not only of long-term psychotherapy, but also of other modalities of therapy, including focal therapy, group therapy, and behavior modification therapy, to delineate more clearly the areas of effectiveness of each type. As noted before, mixtures of modalities should also be carefully studied. Criteria should be developed to determine when to shift from one treatment modality to another, that is, how to decide when a treatment strategy has failed and what should be tried next.

Conclusion

We are aware that the picture we have evoked from our crystal ball of the future psychotherapist and the future of psychotherapy is, in some respects, sobering, but in other respects, encouraging, depending in part on whose interests are being considered. In sum, the future psychotherapist, in this picture, is likely to be a woman with a degree other than medical, doing brief, most often group, psychotherapy within a managed care setting. A larger segment of society will have the opportunity to obtain some brief psychiatric and possibly psychotherapeutic help, while long-term psychotherapy will be restricted to the very few who are wealthy enough to afford it outside of the managed health-care system. Psychiatric education and diagnostic categories are likely to be altered in keeping with the prevailing patterns of practice at the time.

Not only psychiatrists, but all mental health professionals, have an obligation to be aware of what profound transformations the current trends portend. We must be able to adapt to those unavoidable ones dictated by socioeconomic necessity, and must work to forestall or reshape those that will entail damage both to society and science.

References

Adler G: Transitional phenomena, projective identification, and the essential ambiguity of the psychoanalytic situation. Psychoanalytic Quarterly 58:81–104, 1989

Arnold R: Women in the New Zealand teaching profession 1877–1920: a comparative perspective. New Zealand Journal of Educational Studies 20:70–81, 1985

Association of American Medical Colleges: Women in Medicine Statistics. Washington, DC, Association of American Medical Colleges (One Dupont Circle, N.W. Washington, D.C. 20036), February, 1987

Baker T: Big Strides for Women. American Medical News. September 11, 1987

Barrett JE, Rose RM: Mental Disorders in the Community: Progress and Challenge. Proceedings of the 75th Annual Meeting of the American Psychopathological Association, New York City, February 28–March 2, 1985. New York, NY, Guilford, 1986

Bellah RN, Madsen R, Sullivan WN, et al: Habits of the Heart: Individualism and Commitment in American Life. New York, NY, Harper & Row, 1986

Bennett M: The greening of the HMO: implications for prepaid psychiatry. American Journal of Psychiatry 145:1544–1550, 1988

Bickel J: Women in medical education: a status report. New England Journal of Medicine 319:1579–1588, 1988

Borus J: How will new practice settings change psychiatry? in The Future of Psychiatry as a Medical Specialty. Edited by Yager J. Washington, DC, American Psychiatric Press, 1989

Brown S, Dolan B, Painton P: Do you want to die? Time Magazine. May 28, 1990, p 59

Dezell M: The meter's running on mental health. The Boston Phoenix, December 9, p 4, 1988

Directory of the American Psychological Association, 1989 Edition. "989 APA Membership Statistics," Washington, DC, Vol I, p vii

Einthoven A, Kronick R: A consumer-choice health plan for the 1990s: universal health insurance in a system designed to promote quality and economy. New England Journal of Medicine 320:29–37, 1989

Evelyn R: Large employers begin to flee HMOs. The Psychiatric Times 4:1,2,22, June 1987

Feigelson E, Friedman S: The decline of psychiatric career choice: possible role of increasing clinical psychology programs? Journal of Psychiatric Education 8:142–148, 1984

Fenton W: Professional activities of psychiatrists, in The Nation's Psychiatrists: 1983 Survey. Washington, DC, American Psychiatric Press, 1987

Fenton WS, Robinowitz CB, Leaf PJ: Male and female psychiatrists and their patients. American Journal of Psychiatry 144:358–361, 1987

Frank E, Kupfer D, Perel J: Early recurrence in unipolar depression. Archives of General Psychiatry 46:397–400, 1989

GAP Committee on Therapy. Psychotherapy and Its Financial Feasibility in the National Health Care System. New York, Group for the Advancement of Psychiatry, 1978

GAP Committee on Therapy: Teaching Psychotherapy in Contemporary Psychiatric Residency Training. New York, Group for the Advancement of Psychiatry, 1986

GAP Committee on Governmental Agencies: New Roles for Changing Times. New York, Group for the Advancement of Psychiatry, 1987

Ginzburg E: The monetarization of medical care. New England Journal of Medicine 310:1162–1165, 1984

Ginzburg E:. For profit medicine—a reassessment. New England Journal of Medicine 319:757–761, 1988

Goleman D: Social workers vault into a leading role in psychotherapy. New York Times, April 30, 1985, pp C1, C9

Goleman D: New paths to mental health puts strains on some healers. New York Times, May 17, 1990, p B12

Gurevitz H: Psychiatry and preferred provider organizations. Psychiatric Annals 14:342–349, 1984

Holden H, Blose J: Changes in health care costs and utilization associated with mental health treatment. Hospital and Community Psychiatry 38:1066–1080, 1987

Hsiao WC, Braun P, Dunn D, et al: Resource-based relative values. Journal of the American Medical Association 260:2347–2353, 1988

Kandel E: Genes, nerve cells, and the remembrance of things past. Journal of Neuropsychiatry and Clinical Neurosciences 1:103–125, 1989

Kantrowitz JL, Katz AL, Paolitto F, et al: Affect availability, tolerance, complexity, and modulation in psychoanalysis: followup of a longitudinal prospective study. Journal of the American Psychoanalytic Association 34:529–559, 1986

Kantrowitz JL, Katz AL, Paolitto F, et al: Changes in the level and quality of object relations in psychoanalysis: followup of a longitudinal prospective study. Journal of the American Psychoanalytic Association 35:23–46, 1987

Kubie L: Need for a new subdiscipline in the medical profession. Archives of Neurology and Psychiatry 78:283–293, 1957

Langsley D, Yager J: The definition of a psychiatrist: eight years later. American Journal of Psychiatry 145:469–475, 1988

Levin B, Glasser G: A national survey of prepaid mental health services. Hospital and Community Psychiatry 35:350–355, 1984

Luborsky L, Crits-Christoph P, Mintz J, et al: Who Will Benefit From Psychotherapy? Predicting Therapeutic Outcomes. New York, Basic Books, 1988

Manderscheid R, Barrett S (eds): Mental Health, United States, 1987. Rockville, MD, U.S. Department of Health and Human Services, National Institute of Mental Health, 1987

Michels R, Eth S: Ethical issues in psychiatric research on communities: a case study of the community mental health center program, in Ethical Issues in Epidemiological Research, Vol. 7. Edited by Tancredi L. New Brunswick, NJ, Rutgers University Press, 1986

Miller I, Norman W, Keitner G: Cognitive-behavioral treatment of depressed inpatients. American Journal of Psychiatry 146:1274–1279, 1989

Morrison A: Shame, the Underside of Narcissism. Hillsdale, NJ, Analytic Press, 1989

Mumford E, Schlesinger H, Glass G, et al: A new look at evidence about reduced cost of medical utilization following mental health treatment. American Journal of Psychiatry 141:1145–1158, 1984

National Association of Private Psychiatric Hospitals: Surveys on the Impact of Psychiatric Case Management and Managed Care. 1988

Offenkrantz W, Altschul S, Cooper A, et al: Treatment planning and psychodynamic psychiatry, in Treatment Planning in Psychiatry. Edited by Lewis JM, Usdin G. Washington, DC, American Psychiatric Press, 1982, pp 1–41

Open Minds, The Behavioral Health Industry Analyst: Open Minds Study Finds That Psychiatrists Lost Major Market Share in Recent Years. April 11, 1990

Page L: Report notes impact of alternative delivery systems. American Medical News, December 18, 1987, p 12

Richmond A, Brown M: Reimbursement by Medicare for mental health services by general practitioners: clinical, epidemiological, and cost containment implications of the Canadian experience, in Mental Health Service in Primary Settings: Report of a Conference, April 2–3, 1979, Washington, DC. Edited by Baron D, Solomon F. NIMH Mental Health Services Systems Report, 1980, pp 122–130

Robins L, Melzer J, Weissman M, et al: Lifetime prevalence of specific psychiatric disorders in three sites. Archives of General Psychiatry 41:949–958, 1984

Schneider-Braus K: A practical guide to HMO psychiatry. Hospital and Community Psychiatry 38:867–879, 1987

Starr P: The Social Transformation of American Medicine. New York, Basic Books, 1982

Srole L, Langner T, Michael S, et al: Mental Health in the Metropolis: The Midtown Study. New York, McGraw-Hill, 1962

Winslow R: Spending to cut mental-health costs. The Wall Street Journal. December 13, 1989, p 1B

Wallerstein R: Forty-Two Lives in Treatment: A Study of Psychoanalysis and Psychotherapy. New York, Guilford, 1986

Zimet C: The mental health care revolution. American Psychologist 44:703–709, 1989

GAP Committees and Membership

Committee on Adolescence

Warren J. Gadpaille, Denver, CO, *Chairperson*
Hector R. Bird, New York, NY
Ian A. Canino, New York, NY
Michael G. Kalogerakis, New York, NY
Paulina F. Kernberg, New York, NY
Clarice J. Kestenbaum, New York, NY
Richard C. Marohn, Chicago, IL
Silvio J. Onesti, Jr., Belmont, MA

Committee on Aging

Gene D. Cohen, Washington, DC, *Chairperson*
Karen Blank, West Hartford, CT
Eric D. Caine, Rochester, NY
Charles M. Gaitz, Houston, TX
Ira R. Katz, Philadelphia, PA
Andrew F. Leuchter, Los Angeles, CA
Gabe J. Maletta, Minneapolis, MN
Richard A. Margolin, Nashville, TN
George H. Pollock, Chicago, IL
Kenneth M. Sakauye, New Orleans, LA
Charles A. Shamoian, Larchmont, NY
F. Conyers Thompson, Jr., Atlanta, GA

Committee on Alcoholism and the Addictions

Joseph Westermeyer, Minneapolis, MN, *Chairperson*
Margaret H. Bean-Bayog, Lexington, MA
Susan J. Blumenthal, Washington, DC
Richard J. Frances, Newark, NJ
Marc Galanter, New York, NY
Edward J. Khantzian, Haverhill, MA
Earl A. Loomis, Jr., Augusta, GA
Sheldon I. Miller, Newark, NJ
Robert B. Millman, New York, NY
Steven M. Mirin, Belmont, MA
Edgar P. Nace, Dallas, TX
Norman L. Paul, Lexington, MA
Peter Steinglass, Washington, DC
John S. Tamerin, Greenwich, CT

Committee on Child Psychiatry

Peter E. Tanguay, Los Angeles, CA, *Chairperson*
James M. Bell, Canaan, NY
Harlow Donald Dunton, New York, NY
Joseph Fischhoff, Detroit, MI
Joseph M. Green, Madison, WI
John F. McDermott, Jr., Honolulu, HI
David A. Mrazek, Denver, CO
Cynthia R. Pfeffer, White Plains, NY
John Schowalter, New Haven, CT
Theodore Shapiro, New York, NY
Leonore Terr, San Francisco, CA

Committee on College Students

Earle Silber, Chevy Chase, MD, *Chairperson*
Robert L. Arnstein, Hamden, CT
Varda Backus, La Jolla, CA
Harrison P. Eddy, New York, NY
Myron B. Liptzin, Chapel Hill, NC

Malkah Tolpin Notman, Brookline, MA
Gloria C. Onque, Pittsburgh, PA
Elizabeth Aub Reid, Cambridge, MA
Lorraine D. Siggins, New Haven, CT
Tom G. Stauffer, White Plains, NY

Committee on Cultural Psychiatry

Ezra Griffith, New Haven, CT, *Chairperson*
Edward Foulks, New Orleans, LA
Pedro Ruiz, Houston, TX
Ronald Wintrob, Providence, RI
Joe Yamamoto, Los Angeles, CA

Committee on the Family

Herta A. Guttman, Montreal, PQ, *Chairperson*
W. Robert Beavers, Dallas, TX
Ellen M. Berman, Merrion, PA
Lee Combrinck-Graham, Evanston, IL
Ira D. Glick, New York, NY
Frederick Gottlieb, Los Angeles, CA
Henry U. Grunebaum, Cambridge, MA
Ann L. Price, Avon, CT
Lyman C. Wynne, Rochester, NY

Committee on Governmental Agencies

Roger Peele, Washington, DC, *Chairperson*
Mark Blotcky, Dallas, TX
James P. Cattell, San Diego, CA
Thomas L. Clannon, San Francisco, CA
Naomi Heller, Washington, DC
John P.D. Shemo, Charlottesville, VA
William W. Van Stone, Washington, DC

Committee on Handicaps

William H. Sack, Portland, OR, *Chairperson*
Norman R. Bernstein, Cambridge, MA
Meyer S. Gunther, Wilmette, IL
Robert Nesheim, Duluth, MN
Betty J. Pfefferbaum, Norman, OK
William A. Sonis, Philadelphia, PA
Margaret L. Stuber, Los Angeles, CA
George Tarjan, Los Angeles, CA
Thomas G. Webster, Washington, DC
Henry H. Work, Bethesda, MD

Committee on Human Sexuality

Bertram H. Schaffner, New York, NY, *Chairperson*
Paul L. Adams, Galveston, TX
Richard Frieman, New York, NY
Johanna A. Hoffman, Scottsdale, AZ
Joan A. Lang, Galveston, TX
Stuart E. Nichols, New York, NY
Harris B. Peck, New Rochelle, NY
John P. Spiegel, Waltham, MA
Terry S. Stein, East Lansing, MI

Committee on International Relations

Vamik D. Volkan, Charlottesville, VA, *Chairperson*
Robert M. Dorn, El Macero, CA
John S. Kafka, Washington, DC
Otto F. Kernberg, White Plains, NY
John E. Mack, Chestnut Hill, MA
Roy W. Menninger, Topeka, KS
Peter A. Olsson, Houston, TX
Rita R. Rogers, Palos Verdes Estates, CA
Stephen B. Shanfield, San Antonio, TX

Committee on Medical Education

Stephen C. Scheiber, Deerfield, IL, *Chairperson*
Charles M. Culver, Hanover, NH
Steven L. Dubovsky, Denver, CO
Saul I. Harrison, Torrance, CA
David R. Hawkins, Chicago, IL
Harold I. Lief, Philadelphia, PA
Carol Nadelson, Boston, MA
Carolyn B. Robinowitz, Washington, DC
Sidney L. Werkman, Washington, DC
Veva H. Zimmerman, New York, NY

Committee on Mental Health Services

W. Walter Menninger, Topeka, KS, *Chairperson*
Mary Jane England, Roseland, NJ
Robert O. Friedel, Richmond, VA
John M. Hamilton, Columbia, MD
Jose Maria Santiago, Tucson, AZ
Steven S. Sharfstein, Baltimore, MD
Herzl R. Spiro, Milwaukee, WI
William L. Webb, Jr., Hartford, CT
George F. Wilson, Somerville, NJ
Jack A. Wolford, Pittsburgh, PA

Committee on Planning and Marketing

Robert W. Gibson, Towson, MD, *Chairperson*
Allan Beigel, Tucson, AZ
Doyle I. Carson, Dallas, TX
Paul J. Fink, Philadelphia, PA
Robert S. Garber, Longboat Key, FL
Richard K. Goodstein, Belle Mead, NJ
Harvey L. Ruben, New Haven, CT
Melvin Sabshin, Washington, DC
Michael R. Zales, Quechee, VT

Committee on Preventive Psychiatry

Committee on Psychiatry and the Community

Committee on Psychiatry and the Law

Committee on Psychiatry and Religion

Richard C. Lewis, New Haven, CT, *Chairperson*
Naleen N. Andrade, Honolulu, HI
Keith G. Meador, Nashville, TN
Abigail R. Ostow, Belmont, MA
Sally K. Severino, White Plains, NY
Clyde R. Snyder, Fayetteville, NC
Edwin R. Wallace IV, Augusta, GA

Committee on Psychiatry in Industry

Barrie S. Greiff, Newton, MA, *Chairperson*
Peter L. Brill, Radnor, PA
Duane Q. Hagen, St. Louis, MO
R. Edward Huffman, Asheville, NC
Robert Larsen, San Francisco, CA
David E. Morrison, Palatine, IL
David B. Robbins, Chappaqua, NY
Jay B. Rohrlich, New York, NY
Clarence J. Rowe, St. Paul, MN
Jeffrey L. Speller, Cambridge, MA

Committee on Psychopathology

David A. Adler, Boston, MA, *Chairperson*
Jeffrey Berlant, Summit, NJ
John P. Docherty, Nashua, NH
Robert A. Dorwart, Cambridge, MA
Robert E. Drake, Hanover, NH
James M. Ellison, Watertown, MA
Howard H. Goldman, Potomac, MD
Anthony F. Lehman, Baltimore, MD
Kathleen A. Pajer, Pittsburgh, PA
Samuel G. Siris, Glen Oaks, NY

Committee on Public Education

Steven E. Katz, New York, NY, *Chairperson*
Jack W. Bonner, III, Asheville, NC
John Donnelly, Hartford, CT
Jeffrey L. Geller, Worcester, MA
Keith H. Johansen, Dallas, TX
Elise K. Richman, Scarsdale, NY
Boris G. Rifkin, Branford, CT
Andrew E. Slaby, Summit, NJ
Robert A. Solow, Los Angeles, CA
Calvin R. Sumner, Buckhannon, WV

Committee on Research

Robert Cancro, New York, NY, *Chairperson*
Jack A. Grebb, New York, NY
John H. Greist, Madison, WI
Jerry M. Lewis, Dallas, TX
John G. Looney, Durham, NC
Sidney Malitz, New York, NY
Zebulon Taintor, New York, NY

Committee on Social Issues

Ian E. Alger, New York, NY, *Chairperson*
William R. Beardslee, Waban, MA
Judith H. Gold, Halifax, N.S.
Roderic Gorney, Los Angeles, CA
Martha J. Kirkpatrick, Los Angeles, CA
Perry Ottenberg, Philadelphia, PA
Kendon W. Smith, Pearl River, NY

Committee on Therapeutic Care

Donald W. Hammersley, Washington, DC, *Chairperson*
Bernard Bandler, Cambridge, MA

Thomas E. Curtis, Chapel Hill, NC
Donald C. Fidler, Morgantown, WV
William B. Hunter, III, Albuquerque, NM
Roberto L. Jimenez, San Antonio, TX
Milton Kramer, Cincinnati, OH
Theodore Nadelson, Jamaica Plain, MA
William W. Richards, Anchorage, AK

Committee on Therapy

Allen D. Rosenblatt, La Jolla, CA, *Chairperson*
Gerald Adler, Boston, MA
Jules R. Bemporad, Boston, MA
Eugene B. Feigelson, Brooklyn, NY
Robert Michels, New York, NY
Andrew P. Morrison, Cambridge, MA
William C. Offenkrantz, Carefree, AZ

Contributing Members

Gene Abroms, Ardmore, PA
Carlos C. Alden, Jr., Buffalo, NY
Kenneth Z. Altshuler, Dallas, TX
Francis F. Barnes, Washington, DC
Spencer Bayles, Houston, TX
C. Christian Beels, New York, NY
Elissa P. Benedek, Ann Arbor, MI
Sidney Berman, Washington, DC
H. Keith H. Brodie, Durham, NC
Charles M. Bryant, San Francisco, CA
Ewald W. Busse, Durham, NC
Robert N. Butler, New York, NY
Eugene M. Caffey, Jr., Bowie, MD
Robert J. Campbell, New York, NY
Ian L.W. Clancey, Maitland, Ont.
Sanford I. Cohen, Coral Gables, FL
James S. Eaton, Jr., Washington, DC
Lloyd C. Elam, Nashville, TN

Joseph T. English, New York, NY
Louis C. English, Pomona, NY
Sherman C. Feinstein, Highland Park, IL
Archie R. Foley, New York, NY
Sidney Furst, Bronx, NY
Henry J. Gault, Highland Park, IL
Alexander Gralnick, Port Chester, NY
Milton Greenblatt, Sylmar, CA
Lawrence F. Greenleigh, Los Angeles, CA
Stanley I. Greenspan, Bethesda, MD
Jon E. Gudeman, Milwaukee, WI
Stanley Hammons, Lexington, KY
William Hetznecker, Merion Station, PA
J. Cotter Hirschberg, Topeka, KS
Johanna Hoffman, Scottsdale, AZ
Jay Katz, New Haven, CT
James A. Knight, New Orleans, LA
Othilda M. Krug, Cincinnati, OH
Judith Landau-Stanton, Rochester, NY
Alan I. Levenson, Tucson, AZ
Ruth W. Lidz, Woodbridge, CT
Orlando B. Lightfoot, Boston, MA
Norman L. Loux, Sellersville, PA
Albert J. Lubin, Woodside, CA
John A. MacLeod, Cincinnati, OH
Charles A. Malone, Barrington, RI
Peter A. Martin, Lake Orion, MI
Ake Mattsson, Charlottesville, VA
Alan A. McLean, Gig Harbor, WA
David Mendell, Houston, TX
Mary E. Mercer, Nyack, NY
Derek Miller, Chicago, IL
Richard D. Morrill, Boston, MA
Robert J. Nathan, Philadelphia, PA
Joseph D. Noshpitz, Washington, DC
Mortimer Ostow, Bronx, NY
Bernard L. Pacella, New York, NY
Herbert Pardes, New York, NY
Marvin E. Perkins, Salem, VA

David N. Ratnavale, Bethesda, MD
Richard E. Renneker, Pacific Palisades, CA
W. Donald Ross, Cincinnati, OH
Loren Roth, Pittsburgh, PA
Donald J. Scherl, Brooklyn, NY
Charles Shagass, Philadelphia, PA
Miles F. Shore, Boston, MA
Albert J. Silverman, Ann Arbor, MI
Benson R. Snyder, Cambridge, MA
David A. Soskis, Bala Cynwyd, PA
Jeanne Spurlock, Washington, DC
Brandt F. Steele, Denver, CO
Alan A. Stone, Cambridge, MA
Perry C. Talkington, Dallas, TX
Bryce Templeton, Philadelphia, PA
Prescott W. Thompson, Portland, OR
John A. Turner, San Francisco, CA
Gene L. Usdin, New Orleans, LA
Kenneth N. Vogtsberger, San Antonio, TX
Andrew S. Watson, Ann Arbor, MI
Joseph B. Wheelwright, Kentfield, CA
Robert L. Williams, Houston, TX
Paul Tyler Wilson, Bethesda, MD
Sherwyn M. Woods, Los Angeles, CA
Kent A. Zimmerman, Menlo Park, CA
Howard Zonana, New Haven, CT

Life Members

C. Knight Aldrich, Charlottesville, VA
Robert L. Arnstein, Hamden, CT
Bernard Bandler, Cambridge, MA
Walter E. Barton, Hartland, VT
Viola W. Bernard, New York, NY
Henry W. Brosin, Tucson, AZ
John Donnelly, Hartford, CT
Merrill T. Eaton, Omaha, NE
O. Spurgeon English, Narberth, PA
Stephen Fleck, New Haven, CT

Jerome Frank, Baltimore, MD
Robert S. Garber, Longboat Key, FL
Robert I. Gibson, Towson, MD
Margaret M. Lawrence, Pomona, NY
Jerry M. Lewis, Dallas, TX
Harold I. Lief, Philadelphia, PA
Judd Marmor, Los Angeles, CA
Herbert C. Modlin, Topeka, KS
John C. Nemiah, Hanover, NH
William Offenkrantz, Carefree, NM
Mabel Ross, Sun City, AZ
Julius Schreiber, Washington, DC
Robert E. Switzer, Dunn Loring, VA
George Tarjan, Los Angeles, CA
Jack A. Wolford, Pittsburgh, PA
Henry H. Work, Bethesda, MD

Board of Directors

Officers

President
Allan Beigel
P.O. Box 43460
Tucson, AZ 85733

President-Elect
Charles Wilkinson,
600 E. 22nd Street
Kansas City, MO 64108

Secretary
Doyle I. Carson
Timberlawn Psychiatric Hospital
P.O. Box 151489
Dallas, TX 75315-1489

Treasurer
Jack W. Bonner, III
Highland Hospital
P.O. Box 1101
Asheville, NC 28802

Board Members
Judith Gold
Harvey L. Ruben
Pedro Ruiz
John Schowalter

Past Presidents
*William C. Menninger 1946-51
Jack R. Ewalt 1951-53
Walter E. Barton 1953-55
*Sol W. Ginsburg 1955-57
*Dana L. Farnsworth 1957-59
*Marion E. Kenworthy 1959-61
Henry W. Brosin 1961-63
*Leo H. Bartemeier 1963-65
Robert S. Garber 1965-67
Herbert C. Modlin 1967-69
John Donnelly 1969-71
George Tarjan 1971-73
Judd Marmor 1973-75
John C. Nemiah 1975-77
Jack A. Wolford 1977-79
Robert W. Gibson 1979-81
*Jack Weinberg 1981-82
Henry H. Work 1982-85
Michael R. Zales 1985-87
Jerry M. Lewis 1987-89
Carolyn Robinowitz 1989-91

*deceased

Smith Kline Beckman Corporation
Tappanz Foundation, Inc.
The Upjohn Company
van American Foundation, Inc.
Wyeth Laboratories
Mr. and Mrs. William A. Zales